TEETH

WHITENING

Teeth Whitening

How To Whiten Teeth Easily

Monica Harper

The information provided in this book is designed to provide helpful information on the subjects discussed. This book is not meant to be used, nor should it be used, to diagnose or treat any medical condition. For diagnosis or treatment of any medical problem, consult your own physician. The publisher and author are not responsible for any specific health or allergy needs that may require medical supervision and are not liable for any damages or negative consequences from any treatment, action, application or preparation, to any person reading or following the information in this book. References are provided for informational purposes only and do not constitute endorsement of any websites or other sources. Readers should be aware that the websites listed in this book may change.

Table of Content

Is Teeth Whitening For Everyone?

The teeth whitening industry has been booming in recent years and those who are considering it have plenty of choices when it comes to whitening their teeth. However, there are many people who are unaware of teeth whitening.

Do you need them? What causes yellow teeth? Are people blessed with them? There are many questions about this condition and many people fail to address them before considering the teeth whitening process.

Those people who have either brown or yellow stained teeth are very self-conscious of their condition as their family or friends might have mentioned about this to them. It feels very uncomfortable when other people are constantly looking at our teeth and finding fault with them.

There are various reasons as to why you are suffering from this condition. However, the most often cited reason for this is because of tobacco and tartar that is build up from smoking or poor oral health.

Many people who have this yellow teeth condition feel extremely uncomfortable that their teeth are yellow or stained. Nicotine isn't the only terrible habit which causes staining to the enamel.

Among the other things which cause problems to your teeth as well include red wine, caffeine, gravy and several other causes. This depends on the frequency of use in which you place your teeth on but with the right treatment, then you don't have to worry.

Teeth whitening procedure won't improve your health over the long term. It is a cosmetic process which simply lightens the stains on your teeth with proper treatment. However, to first treat this condition, we would first need to understand why your teeth are stained and yellow.

Most of the time, this condition is when you drink certain drinks such as coffee, tea, red wine or cola. Smoking is also one of the chief causes for this condition. There are pores on the enamel of your teeth. They hold onto stains and normal daily brushing wouldn't be sufficient if you want to remove the stains to give you a brighter white look from your beautiful teeth.

Besides stains, discoloration could also occur when someone ages. The stains would appear over a period of time from the inside as there is an excess fluoride and possibly medication has harmed your teeth. Tooth whitening deals with the stains on the outside of your teeth and should be done on a consistent basis.

More customers are experiencing different benefits from teeth whitening. They may have experience the benefits from following the procedure either from teeth whitening specialists or dentists. As such, these procedures are becoming increasingly more popular as customers seek these treatments. Customers look for more experienced teeth professionals in order to help them with such a treatment

In many cases, teeth whitening treatments lasts only as long as your bad habits are still apparent. As such, if you continue smoking or drinking coffee, the staining would only return in about six to nine months after treatment. It could last up to eighteen months if proper care and attention is given.

One of the most popular options is professional laser teeth whitening. The customer should consider visiting their professional dentist to ensure that there are any works that you should do before considering teeth whitening.

Many people strive for a bright white smile. Hollywood superstars and famous celebrities are known for having glowing white teeth with their beautiful smile. As such, many people want whiter teeth also. This has made the teeth whitening industry a booming industry.

Like many beauty industries that have seen massive growth throughout the years, the teeth whitening industry has seen similar growth as well. This is mainly because people are looking to look more glamorous and beautiful; and nothing is more important than having a beautiful set of teeth. This applies to both sexes.

Our society has placed a lot of emphasis on looking good and all of us want to look good. Many of the famous people have white teeth with a beautiful smile. To have beautiful teeth, it depends mainly on the two veneers, which is a type of plastic coating which you apply on the top layer of your teeth. This gives a dynamic white tooth which is consistent across your teeth.

This book would show you how you can have whiter teeth, not only using modern-day surgery but natural methods as well. Read on!

How To Achieve the Perfect Smile

Everyone wants to have the perfect smile that celebrities have. You flip through magazines and see those famous people who just seem to have the killer smile. To have a killer smile, the most important thing is to have sparkling, shiny and bright teeth.

Nowadays, many people are spending a lot of money just to have whiter teeth. They want to make the best use of the teeth whitening treatments and undergo the proper procedures to achieve the perfect white teeth and many people have spent up to tens of thousands just to ensure they have beautiful teeth.

Teeth-whitening is an extremely effective procedure if you want to lighten the color of your teeth without taking away anything on the tooth surface. This wouldn't completely whiten the whole teeth, but would lighten the existing color of your teeth with ease.

There are only very few people in this world who are truly blessed with pearly white teeth and for most people, our teeth would normally become discolored as we grow up. This is a normal thing because aging plays a factor as well. Besides that, our teeth would be stained on the outer part because of the food and drinks.

Drinks like tea, coffee, blackcurrant and red wine would affect severely on the color of your teeth. Another major cause of teeth discoloration is when someone smokes excessively. Smoking has certain chemicals which would stick to the teeth and make your teeth yellow and ugly.

Many people would encounter a certain staining beneath the surface which is normally caused when there are tiny cracks in the teeth or when you have certain antibiotics which absorb the stains.

Among the most common method of whitening your teeth is bleaching. However, make sure that you first visit your doctor for advice beforehand to ensure that this is the a teeth whitening procedure for you that would suit you.

Bleaching is done by simply placing a gel or rubber to shield the soft tissue of your gums. From there, the whitening product is applied on your teeth by a special tray which shapes onto your mouth, similarly to a gum shell.

This teeth whitening product would normally contain carbamide proxide and hydrogen peroxide as the 'active ingredients'. As these ingredients break down, oxygen enters your teeth enamel and makes the color of your teeth lighter. Most general treatment plans for bleaching would last for around three to four weeks.

Those who want to go under this treatment would need at least three visits to the dentist. On the very first visit, the dentist would create a mouth-guard and take an impression of it.

The moment treatment has started; you should continue doing it at home. Generally, you would need to apply this teeth whitening product over a period of four weeks, for a minimum of 30 minutes at a time.

Most of the best teeth whitening products could be applied for up to several hours at a time. This treatment could be done even while you are deep asleep. Ideally, if you want to look for good results, it could be attained as quickly as in a week.

Another very common teeth whitening procedure is known as laser whitening or also known as 'power whitening'. It may be expensive, but it is incredibly effective. Many famous celebrities have been known to go for this procedure and it is known as the best teeth whitening method.

In this process, a rubber dam is gently placed over the teeth in order to shield your gums. From here, the whitening product is gently painted onto your teeth. A laser would be used to stimulate the chemical and the light would boost the chemical reaction of the bleaching product. As such, the color change could be attained more rapidly.

Many dentists believe that the results that you will get from laser whitening treatments are good. According to results, your teeth would be up to six shades lighter.

However, this is a procedure which not everyone would have a chance to undergo. You would first need to get a checkup from your dentist. This is to ensure that you are fit for this treatment. This is a short procedure that would normally be done in an hour.

This is a very powerful procedure and the effects of them could last for up to three years depending on your staining. The dentist would advise you not to smoke, drink or eat any products which could cause a stain on your teeth as they could create serious consequences.

Some people who undergo this procedure may find that their teeth are vulnerable to cold after undergoing it. However, don't worry as these symptoms would go away after a few days.

These two procedures are the most popular and best teeth whitening methods available in the market. They may be very costly, but they would have tremendous positive effect on your teeth, and thus your life. Through these procedures, you would flash everyone that perfect smile that you yearn.

Teeth Whitening Products And Methods

Our teeth is one of the most important feature of your face, regardless of whether you are a men or women. It is important to have a straight set of teeth and dazzling smile, as one can win multiple 'battles' by merely having a killer smile.

It is very common for you to hear nowadays that having a good external appearance play a very important role in ensuring that you have better personal relationship. It may be a harsh truth, but it is still something that is very common in the workplace or in the business world.

In the market these days, there are plenty of products and methods that would help you achieve this purpose. It is simply a common method of whitening your teeth to ensure that they are brighter and cleaner.

A very popular technique is known as dental bleaching and could be used to ensure that your teeth are in better shape than original. The discolouring of your teeth may be due to several reasons. Teeth staining could be due to several reasons like coffee, tobacco and other food particles.

To ensure that you can whiten your teeth successfully, there are certain elements like tetracycline which help restore the enamel of the teeth. The moment your enamel of your teeth is restored, you teeth would become whiter over a period of time. You should take good care of your teeth to ensure that they look dazzling and sparkling for a longer period. Ensure that you brush properly to ensure that the natural lustre of your teeth is intact.

Besides that, the colour and shine of your teeth could be hampered due to eating food which is either too hot or cold as well. Oxidizing agents these days are looking for the perfect method of restoring the colour and shine on your teeth. Carbamide peroxide and hydrogen peroxide are excellent oxidizing agents.

However, these kinds of treatments are temporary and would wither away after a period of time. Besides that, there are also several reasons why it withers over time. You need to ensure that you take proper care so that the treatments are not of waste and your teeth stay pretty.

The teeth bleaching would give a new shine and colour and gives the person more confidence. Without a doubt, a more beautiful set of teeth gives you a more stunning face. It is a sign that the person takes good care of themselves. Therefore, it is very important to take good care of your teeth and perform some of those treatments.

The Cost of Teeth Whitening

It doesn't matter if you want a nicer smile for your prom night or simply self-conscious because you have yellow teeth from drinking coffee, whitening remedies would only brighten your smile. From there, you can learn to boost your confidence. Nothing beats having a wonderful smile to light up the room.

In this chapter, you would learn about the general information about the nature of teeth whitening, its different categories, techniques and costs of each method.

Simply put, teeth whitening is an industry under the field of cosmetic dentistry. This process would eliminate stains and discoloration of your teeth due to tea, smoking, coffee and other lifestyle activities. Besides that, whitening could only lighten up other usual teeth pigmentations.

The success of the teeth whitening treatment depends a great deal on the severity and nature of the stains, together with teeth discoloration. Stains due to smoking, coffee or tea would affect your teeth to about four to five shades.

Discoloration due to antibiotics and heredity factors could also lighten between two to three shades after the whitening treatments. Generally put, there are two categories of teeth whitening remedies.

The first one is professional whitening systems. This procedure is normally performed by dentists with whitening gels and lasers to activate the solution. This procedure is normally done inside a dental clinic.

The second category is home-based teeth whitening remedy. This can be done in-between your appointments of professional treatments using whitening kits and tray-based whitening techniques. These are simply home-made remedies made from your kitchen and medicine items. These applications are done from and based on the frequency recommended by dentists or based on the products' instructions.

Without a doubt, your teeth would be much brighter after you use these teeth whitening methods, However, there are various over the counter whitening solutions, do-it yourself or home-made whitening solutions. But before you try any of those, be sure to consult a dentist first as it would help validate the claims made by these remedies. Many of those claims are true, but those situation may be different for different people.

Besides the available time and patient's temperament, you would also need to consider the cost of whitening your teeth.

The cost of teeth whitening depends a lot on the teeth whitening method you want to employ.

Generally, costs of in-office dental whitening methods are between the price range of $500 to $2000. Home-based bleaching trays which are customized by a dentist would meanwhile cost between $100 to $300. Very often, using home-made solutions are inexpensive. Paint whiteners are cheaper and could cost for as low as $50, depending on which country you are in.

There are various questions when it comes to whether you should whiten your teeth. There are various advantages of disadvantages to teeth whitening that depends on the individual.

Nevertheless, the application of any method on the surface of your teeth would bring about brighter teeth and a brighter smile. The amount of time needed before you achieve the wanted result varies, but it is something that is worth being patient for.

Generally, professional techniques would have relatively faster results compares to over-the-counter whitening paints and home-made remedies. It makes sense because professional techniques have faster results.

However, it should be known that peroxide-based gels which are used in the teeth whitening procedure would make the teeth become temporarily sensitive to hot and cold food or drinks. In more severe cases, it would even be affected when exposed to air. Oversensitivity in your gums can also be caused by trays for whitening which are customized by dentists.

An important note to consider is that certain whitening kits which are bought without the recommended prescription would tear down and make the teeth's enamel thinner. This exposes the dentin which makes it severely coloured. These things would add up the cost of having the procedure.

Removing Both Internal And External Stains

When you have stains on your teeth, they are a sign that your teeth aren't very healthy. Your teeth should be taken good care of as they are an asset not only to the looks of a person but also a reflection of your personality. Without a doubt, it is very important to take good care of your teeth to ensure they are healthy.

There are common discoloration of your teeth and they could be internal or external.

The defects that are internal and external are due to various reasons.

Internal reasons could be due to the use of substances like alcohol or tobacco. External reasons may be due to improper care. Besides that, there are also many other reasons why someone would have unpolished and discoloured teeth.

If the discolouring of your teeth is external, it could be easily removed through methods such as bleaching and whitening treatments. These help restore your teeth's enamel and ensure that it goes back to the original colour.

There are also simple and easy solutions which one can use to improve your teeth's colour and ensure that it returns to its natural lustre and shine. The shine and colour of your teeth could be easily improved to a greater level with the use of bleaches and colours. They would greatly uplift a person's confidence when their teeth are in good shape and colour.

However, if the stains on your teeth are internal, there are different forms of treatment. If the stains are from the inside, there are different procedures that should be followed to remove them. These stains could be hidden with the help of root canal or other more complicated procedures.

Generally speaking, the higher the concentration of the whitener, the more effective it is. The better the bleaching is done, the longer it stays. This is an incredibly way of bringing the natural colour and shine of the teeth.

This is the general method of how the stains are removed and to make your teeth more better looking. The teeth can be capped and the colour would look better as well.

Besides that, there is a sort of gel that could be used to bleach the teeth. You could also try home bleaching kits which can be done from the comfort of your home to remove the stains.

Disadvantages Of Teeth Whitening Treatments

From the previous chapters, it is clear that having a perfect smile is incredibly important. The beauty of your smile would be marred if your teeth is discoloured.

Although they are various treatments to ensure your teeth is whiter, they should be treated with caution. The teeth could be kept safe from spoiling and from being discoloured with proper habits. Treatments are split into organic and chemical treatments.

Certain treatments could be used to ensure that your teeth turn out to a better colour. They may sometimes spoil your teeth and make them weaker from the inside. They would sometimes wither the natural enamel of the teeth and this makes them weaker permanently and more prone to ailments.

They may also damage your teeth sometimes. There has been many cases where your teeth have been so permanently discoloured if the amount of chemicals used in the bleaches is not in the right mixture.

Although there are clear disadvantages of teeth whitening treatments, you should realize that there are various benefits if used right.

You need to choose the right product.

Visiting a professional dentist is also very important. Go for the best products in the market. Look for the most genuine of dentists to ensure that your teeth are healthy.

Teeth Whitening Surgery

Teeth whitening surgery is one the best, if not the best method of ensuring that the health of your teeth is bettered and your appearance improved.

There are certain teeth whitening surgeries that make your teeth look better over time. Generally put, teeth are the pearls that are used for the beautification of your face.

These teeth whitening procedures could help restore the beauty of your teeth and they are incredibly effective for the health and clarity of your teeth. There has been a lot of development in the dental industry for teeth whitening surgery.

Besides this, there are also certain more complicated treatments that could be followed by simply whitening your teeth. However, one should always consult a dentist for a professional opinion.

Before choosing your dentist, you need to ensure that the doctor is reputable and professional. Ask from your close ones or simply surf the internet to find a reputable doctor around your area. Read the reviews to check that he or she has the experience in teeth whitening.

A good dentist would be able to help prescribe you with the right treatment and the proper teeth whitening procedures. Professional dentist who have a long history of performing teeth whitening surgery is a great choice to ensure that they are able to give you the right advice.

With this treatment, your teeth could be greatly improved to a great level. This would greatly improve a person's smile and self-esteem.

After performing this surgery, it would definitely improve a person's self-esteem and make them feel better. Before this surgery, you need to ensure that your dental and medical history is clarified with your dentist first.

As such, if you are looking for a good dentist to help you with this procedure, you need to find a good dentist and make it a point to take proper care of your teeth.

Natural Whitening Methods And Cosmetic Treatments

Your teeth are an important asset of your face. There are many wonderful gifts that are blessed on beautiful people, and teeth are an important feature.

You need to take good care of your teeth to ensure that they are healthy and sparkling for a long time. There are many things which can easily damage the shine and lustre of your teeth.

The responsibility of taking care of your teeth lies in you. You must ensure that your teeth are free from infections. There are other methods such as chemical and natural methods which could be used to ensure that your teeth is safe and healthy.

Natural methods are simple methods such as rubbing lime and salt onto your teeth before brushing them. This is a very popular natural method of cleaning your teeth.

Besides that, the teeth could be massaged with guava leaves and it is also a great method of cleaning the teeth from the stains. Other methods include using cotton soaked in baking soda. Strawberries can also be used to clean the teeth of certain impurities.

Besides that, one should also use toothpastes which have a higher amount of fluoride content. This makes your teeth white and removes the yellow-ness.

A great practice to ensure that your mouth is not yellow in the future is to constantly gargle your mouth after every meal you eat. This would ensure that your mouth is fresh and clean from food practices that would stick in corners of your teeth and cause painful infections.

Besides these natural methods, there are also chemical methods which would help as well. There are a number of teeth whitening treatments which are chemical-based. They are incredibly effective and can make a person's smile change greatly.

Laser treatments can be done and there are also cosmetic surgeries which can be done to improve both the colour and texture of your teeth.

Be clear that there are natural and cosmetic methods of teeth whitening. However, one would need to know the health of their teeth before doing any of them. Both are effective in their own right. What you need to do is to choose what is best for yourself.

Chewing Gums For Whiter Teeth

From the past few chapters, I have shared various treatment methods which help make your teeth sparkle for a long period. They may be incredibly effective but they are extremely costly.

Another better option for this is simply by using chewing gums for teeth whitening. There are various chewing gums available in the market that are incredibly effective in helping your teeth restore to it natural colour and improving the enamel of the teeth.

These chewing gums work wonderfully and should be chewed after your meals. They work in a manner which makes the pH levels in your mouth adjust to a more appropriate level.

This would make your teeth fight back the germs which attack on the inside of the teeth each time you eat. If the person is a chronic smoker or coffee addict, these chewing gums are of incredible aid. One doesn't have to spend incredibly amount of money to use complex treatments to get their teeth white with the use of chewing gums.

They are very cheap and could be used more extensively. One just needs to chew these gums after each meal to make their teeth sparkle with the shine and strength.

They are way more convenient compared to the painful and costly visits to the dentist. Many people are also very afraid of the big and crude instruments on the dentist's table.

It is clear that chewing gum is a much feasible option if cost is a main issue for you. If you are someone who is worried of the pain as well, this is also something to consider.

There are abrasives on the chewing gums which help clean the surface of your teeth. Chewing gums would bring the color and help improve the strength of your teeth.

Head to the nearest convenient store or pharmacy to get one today. It may seem like a simple thing, but it's incredibly effective in whitening your teeth over the long run.

Toothpastes For Whiter Teeth

You should take good care of your teeth. Always make sure that your teeth are cleansed and flossed on a regular basis to ensure that there aren't any possible infections which would plaque your teeth and make the weak from the inside.

Your teeth cleaning should be a routine. You should make it a point to have good dental habits. Among the basic one is to brush your teeth twice daily, with toothpaste, of course.

There are quite a number of teeth whitening and polishing toothpastes which are available in the market nowadays. They would help you get better results from brushing your teeth.

Teeth whitening toothpastes are specially formulated and made from herbs which are the most sought after chemicals in the market. They would ensure that your teeth become whiter and your smile is as perfect as it can be

Most teeth whitening formulas consist of a larger value of chloride salts. These salts wouldn't just whiten the teeth but make it strong over a certain period. Your teeth would be sure to sparkle and shine if they are taken good care of.

These toothpastes have various flavors. They not only work well to maintain your teeth's health but also taste yummy, although you should never eat them. Kids would sure to love these toothpastes and ensure that their teeth are strong and dazzling.

You should also use dental flosses regularly to ensure that your teeth look better. However, they aren't a form of treatment. They are merely preventative measures that help to keep away your teeth from dental ailments.

If you follow proper brushing and flossing habits, you can avoid a trip to the dentist. Therefore, it is essential to use the right toothpastes. They come in various flavors like mint, lemon, orange and strawberry that are extracted from herbs. This helps prevent the teeth from having any problem.

If you are an adult, you should make sure that your whole family has great oral hygiene habits. This would help make sure that your family is healthy orally. For parents, developing healthy oral habits while your children are younger is imperative over the long term.

Using Fruits In Teeth Whitening

Your teeth should be sparkling and shiny when you are in a picture. Teeth are more than just for chewing purposes; it also affects your good looks. There has been an incredible amount of teeth whitening treatments that could help improve the color and texture of your teeth.

Home remedies are very helpful for whitening and bleaching your teeth. They help bring them to a better color and improve the health of your enamel.

One great remedy which is natural is strawberries. It is used to improve your teeth. Crushed strawberries could be massaged over the teeth to ensure that they are whitened. It is a natural cleanser and could be used to disinfect. Scrubbing the teeth with it could make it shine even more.

The other alternative to strawberry is lemon. Lemon is a citrus food and is an incredible teeth whitening agent. They are strong and therefore shouldn't be used in a concentrated manner. It should be mixed with other elements to ensure that it comes to a more usable level.

Lemons are a great way to build back the health of your teeth's enamel. This makes them white and sparkling over a long period.

This is the power of using fruits as a remedy for whiter teeth. They are efficient and cheap to use compared to modern medication, which are not only expensive but comes together with certain risks.

Strawberries and lemons are a great way to make sure that your mouth is clean and fresh. This makes the teeth sparkling white. All one needs to do now is to ensure that they take care of their teeth to avoid any more unnecessary visits to the dentist.

Ensure Safety In Teeth Whitening Treatments

Cleanliness should be a priority for your teeth. You should always take good care of ensuring that they retain a natural sheen and shine. There are plenty of treatments nowadays which are available which promises to return your sparkling smile and makes sure that you are confident.

There are so many new and more advanced treatments these days that would magically make your teeth more beautiful and make you pretty in your picture. One thing that I always recommend is to go for natural treatment whenever possible.

In the market, there are many natural or chemical treatments that transform your smile. With your beautiful smile, you are more confident with it and increase your confidence as a person.

The most important is to ensure that you have good oral hygiene habits to ensure that you wouldn't need to take mindless trips to the doctor.

When picking the toothpaste, you shouldn't choose one which has no extra amount of harsh or abrasive chemicals. They would just simply wither away the natural enamel of the teeth. There should be the appropriate amount of Carbamide peroxide gel to ensure it is bleached in the right amount for your teeth.

Another important thing is to have regular dental checkups. Ideally speaking, you should have a dental checkup twice a year. It is important to go for this checkup as having nice teeth is important for your face and personality. Having pearly white teeth would easily boost your confidence.

If you can, choose natural treatments for whitening your teeth. These are simple remedies from fruits like lemons or strawberries. When crushed and applied on the teeth, they become natural cleaning and whitening agent. They are not only cheap but also highly effective.

Safety is important when whitening your teeth. Don't simply try anything without consulting the dentist.

The Importance Of Consulting A Dentist

Having a good dentist is similar to having a magician who could transform your smile, and thus your life. Do you remember those tough times where you were struggling with tooth aches? Those sleepless nights that happened to you due to your aching teeth? The dentist is invaluable in solving all your dental issues and giving you the perfect smile.

It is hard to know what method of treatment is the best for you as there are so many of the in the market nowadays. Anyone who has tried to find for a product would know that you can be easily confused because of it.

From treatments such as laser, braces, bleaching and whitening; all of them can magically transform how your teeth look and how your smile would shape up. The dentist would make sure that all your needs are met and that the right treatment is given to you.

He would look at your teeth to find out the chief cause of the issues you face. A professional one would treat you especially each time you walk into treatment. As such, you should choose the right dentist who is able to communicate with you properly. He would be better equipped to understand your requirements.

Make sure that your dentist know of any complications that you face. These complications may lead to more serious issues. A good dentist would go a long way towards helping your condition. They can prescribe the proper solution.

It is better than trying to try every solution there is in the market and see what suits you. In the long run, seeing a qualified dentist would save you more money over time.

Besides that, you need to be clear about the instructions of the dentist to ensure that you get the best results.

If your teeth bleeds or your gums swell, it could be related to certain serious issues in your teeth. You would need to consult a dentist to ensure that the problem is cured and doesn't get worst.

A dentist isn't as horrible as imagined. Some people are afraid of seeing a dentist because they think that dentists are scary with their tools which are sharp. Treat him as a friend and guide who is here to help you through those issues in your oral health. You would need to get in touch with a professional dentist and he would guide you

with improving your oral condition.

Using Home Remedies To Whiten Your Teeth

Do you want to badly give your smile a makeover? However, you don't have money for it? If so, you could try a do-it-yourself remedy for teeth whitening.

Of course, if you can afford it, you should always go for professional whitening systems. However, if cost is something which is restrictive, you can try using home remedy systems to achieve the similar healthy smile result. What is needed is to simply make a change in the patient's lifestyle that suits the appropriate situation.

In this chapter, we would provide a short appraisal of the teeth whitening system that you could do at the comfort of your home. This would be much cheaper than professional teeth whitening solutions as it would save you a lot of money. However, before trying any of these home-made teeth whitening remedy, you should always consult your doctor although you could easily make your own whitening solutions without spending a fortune.

It may be hard for you to believe but the amount of money you can save is in the hundreds to thousands. As you allocate the required time for applying the tips, you could easily have a white and bright teeth for free. Well, not free, just dirt cheap compared to professional solutions. Most of the ingredients used are the things that could be normally found in your kitchen or medicine kit.

Among the ingredients you need include hydrogen, peroxide, baking soda, cups, spoons and bowls. To make it, mix two/three teaspoons of hydrogen peroxide and two teaspoons of baking soda. Place this mixture in a small bowl. You must ensure that the thickness of the paste is consistent with the normal thickness of toothpaste. For additional taste, you can add a bit of flavour or a little scoop of toothpaste could be easily combined with the homemade paste.

This homemade paste can be used by just using a toothbrush. Leave the mixture on your teeth with the toothbrush for a couple of minutes. Make sure that you don't swallow the paste. If this happens, make sure to drink a lot of water.

After you have brushed the paste on your teeth, you would need to brush it again using normal toothpaste to get rid of the bitter taste of hydrogen peroxide. These remedy could be easily used for those people who are coffee drinkers, smokers and even older people who have stain on their teeth.

If you are someone who has a sensitive oral situation, you need to think about this first before using it. If you have cavities, open sores, gingivitis or gum problems; this paste would make your gums look pale for a short period of time. As said before, always consult a doctor before trying this remedy.

This remedy should be applied on your teeth at least once a week. If you do this excessively, it would be very harming for your teeth. Do-it-yourself teeth whitening systems are great as it is cheap to use but care need to be taken. In summary, for this system to work you need to:

- Be able to allocate a certain amount of time to perform these remedies

- Be capable of performing and following the instructions
- Be patient enough to wait for it to work

Whiten Your Teeth Now

This is a simple and short information on teeth whitening to give you the knowledge about this procedure. This book has given you the essential knowledge needed on the common methods and procedures for teeth whitening.

This book would also helped you get rid of the unnecessary confusion and myths that other people have misled you. From here, hopefully, you are in a better position to understand the importance and power of various teeth whitening solutions.

Whatever method of teeth whitening you settle for, you would need to seek the help of an oral care specialist. I have mentioned this many times in this book for a reason. This is because different patients have different conditions. An oral specialist would be able to determine that.

Even if you seek natural teeth whitening methods, discussing with a dentist is incredibly important. That's what dentists are for. I wish that you get the whitest of teeth in the soonest of time. Good luck!

Resource 1 - Whiten Your Teeth FAST

Do you want…

- **To have whiter and healthier teeth for a longer period of time?**
- To not feel embarrassed next time when you open your mouth?
- **Stop feeling sick and tired of seeing ugly yellow teeth in the mirror each morning?**
- More confidence and fulfilment in your personal relationships?

This is an inexpensive but incredible system that is ***GUARANTEED TO BRING AMAZING RESULTS QUICKLY WHICH LAST FOR YEARS!***

Check out…

http://whiteteeth.wellbeingvalley.com/

Resource 2 - Problem With Teeth Grinding?

Do you have a problem with teeth grinding?

In this guide, you would find a system that is able to:

- Treat teeth grinding naturally and holistically
- Get rid of teeth grinding once and for all
- Stop the pain without the need for pain killers or surgery

Know about your teeth grinding situation and find the right cure. Check out…

http://teethgrinding.wellbeingvalley.com/